CHAMOMILE

MARIAN KIM

CONTENTS

1

PROPERTIES

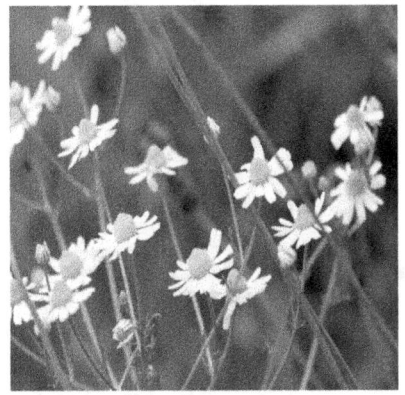

Scientific name: Chamaemelum nobile

Other names: English chamomile

Properties

Analgesic (pain relieving) properties

Anti-inflammatory properties

Antioxidant properties which protect the cells from free radical damage

Antiseptic properties

Emollient (softens and soothes skin)

Moisturizing properties

Skin soothing properties

Anticancer activity against prostate cancer cells

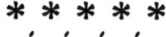

2

USES

Eczema treatment

Chamomile when applied on the skin was found to be about 60% as effective as 0.25% Hydrocortisone cream for the treatment of atopic eczema. N.B. German Chamomile (Matricaria recutita) cream has been proven to be more effective than 0.5% hydrocortisone cream in treating eczema.

Burns

Chamomile is used to treat burns and sunburns.

Minor skin infections

Chamomile is used to treat minor skin infections by bacteria, viruses and fungi since it has antiseptic properties. It is also used for mild rashes.

Wounds

Chamomile is used to manage ulcers and wounds. In fact, some studies suggest that it can cause complete wound healing faster than corticosteroids.

Mouth ulcers treatment

Chamomile infusion is used as a gargle to reduce inflammation in the mouth.

Sore throat reliever

Chamomile infusion is used as a gargle to reduce inflammation in the throat.

Inflammation reducer

Chamomile flower poultices are used to reduce pain and swelling associated with inflammation from infections like abscesses.

Pain reliever

Chamomile is used to reduce the pain of toothaches, earaches and neuralgia (nerve pain).

Digestive aid

Chamomile tea has been used for years as a relaxing tea typically taken after dinner since it also aids digestion and helps a person sleep better. Chamomile is also used for colic, upset stomach, relieving flatulence (gas) and ulcers. It also soothes the stomach and relaxes the muscles that move food through the intestines.

Diarrhea treatment

Chamomile tincture is used to manage summer diarrhea in children. Chamomile tincture is made by mixing 1 cup chamomile flowers with 4 cups water with 12% grain alcohol.

Hypertension treatment

Research suggests that chamomile can lower the systolic blood pressure.

Diabetes treatment

Research suggests that chamomile can lower blood sugar levels and increase storage of glycogen by the liver.

Hemorrhoid treatment

Research suggests that chamomile ointment can improve hemorrhoids. Chamomile infusion can also be added to baths to soothe the ano-genital region. Chamomile tinctures can also be used in sitz baths to reduce the inflammation associated with hemorrhoids.

Anxiety treatment

Chamomile flowers can be placed in boiling water and the vapor inhaled to relieve the symptoms of generalized anxiety disorder. It is also used for depression.

Insomnia treatment

Chamomile has sedative or sleep inducing properties which are useful for managing insomnia or sleeplessness.

Stress management

Chamomile is used for stress management since it has mentally relaxing properties and a soothing aroma. It also relieves tension headaches. Its anti-inflammatory properties protect the body from free radical cell damage during stressful periods when more free radicals are produced.

Acne treatment

Chamomile is soothing to the skin and has anti-inflammatory activity. It also helps in eliminating blackheads by helping open up the pores. Chamomile is also used to manage oily skin since it can eliminate blackheads by helping open up and clean clogged pores.

Dry skin moisturization

Chamomile is used to manage dry skin and cracked nipples since it has soothing and hydrating effects on the skin.

Sensitive skin soothing

Chamomile soothes sensitive skin.

Psoriasis treatment

Chamomile is used to manage psoriasis since it has skin soothing and anti-inflammatory properties. It is also used to manage scalp psoriasis.

Mature skin and prematurely aging skin

Chamomile is used to manage mature and prematurely aging skin since it has antioxidant properties which protect the cells from free radical damage that contributes to the aging process.

Rough skin softener

Chamomile is used for softening hard skin like on the feet

Allergic skin reactions treatment

Chamomile is used for managing allergic skin reactions.

Hay fever treatment

Chamomile is used to treat hay fever.

Under eye circles healer

Chamomile is used to minimize under eye circles.

Inflamed and itchy scalps soother

Chamomile flowers are used to manage scalp psoriasis and soothe inflamed, itchy scalps due to their anti-inflammatory properties.

Damaged hair treatment

Chamomile flowers condition and strengthen dry and damaged hair to prevent breakage.

Alopecia treatment

Chamomile flowers stimulate hair growth and are used to manage thinning hair and hair loss conditions (alopecia).

Dull hair reviver

Chamomile flowers are also used to manage dull hair. They restore shine and enhance natural highlights in blondes.

Arthritis treatment

Chamomile is used to treat arthritis, rheumatism and neuralgia (nerve pain) since it has analgesic or pain relieving properties.

Muscle cramps treatment

Chamomile is used to treat muscle spasms, aches and cramps since it relaxes tense muscles.

PMS treatment

Chamomile is used for premenstrual tension (PMS) and dysmenorrhea or painful periods.

Menopausal symptoms management

Chamomile is used to manage menopausal symptoms.

Menstrual symptoms management

Chamomile is used to manage menstrual disorders.

Surgical scars

Chamomile is also used for surgical scars.

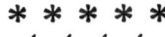

3

SAFETY PRECAUTIONS

1. Avoid chamomile during pregnancy as it may cause miscarriage.

2. Do not use /avoid chamomile if you are allergic to it or allergic to daisy or aster family plants like ragweed, chrysanthemums, marigolds and celery.

3. Do not use /avoid chamomile if you have asthma.

4. Do not use /avoid chamomile if you are driving or operating machines as it may cause drowsiness.

5. Do not use /avoid chamomile if you are taking alcohol.

6. Avoid chamomile if you are scheduled to have surgery or dental procedures within 2 weeks as it may cause bleeding.

4

DRUG INTERACTIONS

1. Do not use/avoid chamomile if you are taking blood thinners like warfarin (coumadin) or antiplatelet drugs like clopidogrel (plavix) or NSAID painkillers like ibuprofen or aspirin as it may cause bleeding since it contains a chemical known as coumarin.

2. Do not use/avoid chamomile if you are taking sedatives or drugs used to treat sleeplessness

3. Do not use/avoid chamomile if you are taking high blood pressure medications as it may lower the blood pressure

4. Do not use/avoid chamomile if you are taking diabetes medications as it can lower the blood sugar.

5

TIPS

Do not use/avoid chamomile if you are taking the following herbs:

1. Garlic

2. Ginkgo biloba

3. Saw palmetto

4. St. John's wort

5. Valerian

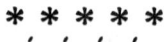

6

HERBAL RECIPES

Chamomile Infused Oil

Equipment
Double boiler

Large glass bowl

Sieve and cheesecloth

Sterilized dark jars

***

Ingredients
16 fl oz. (500 ml) pure vegetable oil such as sweet almond oil or sunflower oil

8 oz. (250 grams) slightly crushed, dry chamomile flowers or 16 oz. (500 grams) slightly bruised fresh chamomile flowers

***

Instructions

1. Place the chamomile flowers and oil in the glass bowl ensuring that the oil covers the herbs. Simmer them in a double boiler for one hour at a temperature of around 120 degrees Fahrenheit (49 degrees Celsius). Do not let the mixture boil. You can repeat this step several times after letting the oils cool to create more concentrated herb infused oils.

2. Strain the mixture through the sieve and cheesecloth into a clean, dark jar ensuring you squeeze out as much oil as you can from the cheesecloth.

3. Label your jars with the manufacturing date, expiry date, herb and oils used.

4. Store your herb infused oils in a cool dark place or in the refrigerator and use them within 3 months.

*****

Chamomile Salve

Equipment

Double boiler

Large glass bowl

Sterilized dark jars or tins

***

Ingredients

8 oz. (250 ml or 1 cup) herb infused vegetable oil (see previous recipe)

1 oz. (30 grams) beeswax

50 drops (2.5 ml or ½ teaspoon) essential oils like lavender essential oil (optional natural fragrance)

***

Instructions

1. Place the beeswax and herb infused oil in the glass bowl and melt them in a double boiler.

2. Once melted remove from the heat source, let them cool before adding the essential oils.

3. Pour the melted oils into the storage jars or tins and allow to cool completely.

4. Store the salves in a cool dark place.

***

Tips

1. Use Roman chamomile essential oil to make the salve more potent for treating eczema.

1. Use German chamomile essential oil to make the salve more potent for treating psoriasis.

2. If you want softer salves you can use less beeswax – for example ¾ oz of beeswax for 1 cup of vegetable oils.

*****

Chamomile Lip Balm

Equipment

Double boiler

Large glass bowl

Lip balm tubes or small jars or tins

***

Ingredients

3 tablespoons herb infused vegetable oil (see recipe above)

1 tablespoon grated beeswax

1 tablespoon shea butter

***

Instructions

1. Place the beeswax, shea butter and herb infused oil in the glass bowl and melt them in a double boiler.

2. Once melted remove from the heat source and pour into lip balm tubes and allow to cool completely.

*****

Chamomile Poultice

Equipment

Cheesecloth or old cotton sheet strips

***

Ingredients

1 tablespoon bruised fresh chamomile flowers or powdered dry chamomile flowers

Boiling water

***

Instructions

1. Add enough boiling water to the chamomile flowers to wet them and make a thick paste.

2. Spoon the herb paste onto the cheesecloth (or bed sheet strips) to make the poultice.

3. To use, apply the poultice to the affected area and cover with another piece of hot, wet cloth. Replace the hot, wet cloth when it cools with another hot one to keep the poultice hot.

*****

Chamomile Tincture

Equipment

Glass jar with tight fitting lid

Dark tincture bottles

Cheesecloth

Labels

***

Ingredients

7 oz (200 gm) of dried chamomile flowers or 14 oz (400 gm) of fresh chamomile flowers

30 oz (1 liter) of 80-100 proof vodka

***

Instructions

1. Fill 1/3 of the glass jar with the chamomile flowers.

2. Add the vodka to completely fill the jar to the top.

3. Seal the jar and label it with the date of preparation and name of herb used.

4. Store the glass jar in a dark place for 6 weeks ensuring that you shake them weekly.

5. After 6 weeks strain out the herbs with a cheesecloth and pour the tincture into dark tincture bottles.

6. Label the tincture bottles with the date and name of herb used.

7. Store your herbal tinctures away from light and heat.

***

Tips

1. You can leave the herbs in the alcohol for up to 6 months if you want to create very strong tinctures.

*****

Chamomile Tea

Equipment

Kettle

Tea cup

***

Ingredients

1 teaspoon of finely crushed or minced chamomile flowers

1 cup of boiling water

Honey to taste (optional)

***

Instructions

1. Put the chamomile flowers in a tea cup, add the boiling water and let it steep while covered for 10 -15 minutes.

3. Add honey (if using) to suit your taste before drinking.

*****

Chamomile Infusion

Equipment

Glass jar with tight fitting lid

***

Ingredients

1 tablespoon dried chamomile flowers or 3 tablespoons fresh chamomile flowers

1 cup boiling water

***

Instructions

1. Place the chamomile flowers in the glass jar and add the boiling water to fill the jar.

2. Close the lid and let the mixture steep for 4 hours to 14 hours (overnight).

3. Strain the herb and the infusion is ready for use.

***

Tips

1. Store the infusion in the refrigerator to lengthen its life.

*****

Chamomile Glycerite

Equipment

Jar with tight fitting lid

Bottle with tight fitting lid

***

Ingredients

1 cup fresh, chopped chamomile or ½ cup dried, crushed chamomile

2 cups vegetable glycerine

***

Instructions

1. Place the chamomile in the jar and pour in the glycerine to fully cover the plant material and fill the jar.

2. Label the jar and store it in a dark place ensuring that you shake it every day.

3. After 4-6 weeks strain the chamomile with a fine sieve or cheese cloth and pour the glycerite into a clean bottle.

4. Label the glycerite and store it in a cool place.

***

Tips

1. Chamomile glycerites can be added to teas to sweeten and flavor them.

*****

Chamomile Compress

Equipment

Large bowl

Clean cloth or cotton balls

***

Ingredients

3 cups Chamomile infusion (see previous recipe)

***

Instructions

1. Pour the chamomile infusion in the bowl.

2. Dip a clean cotton cloth in the infusion and squeeze out the excess fluid while making sure that you do not burn yourself.

3. Apply the chamomile compress on the affected body part.

Tips

1. Chamomile compresses are applied on the stomach to soothe nervous indigestion.

###

ABOUT THE AUTHOR

Marian Kim is an experienced alternative medicine practitioner.

OTHER BOOKS BY THE AUTHOR

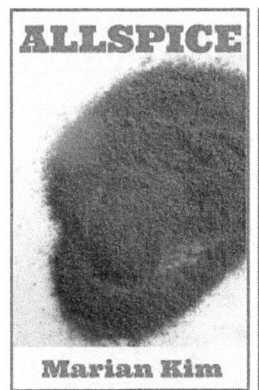

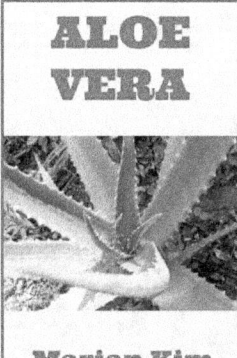

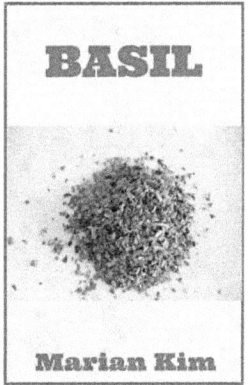

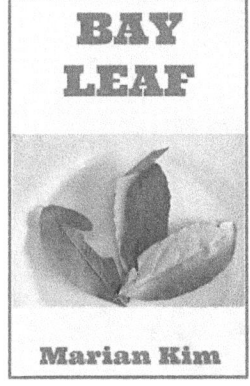

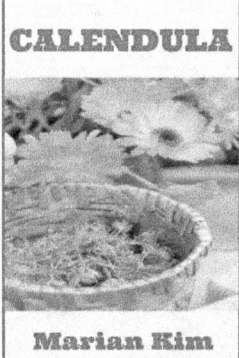

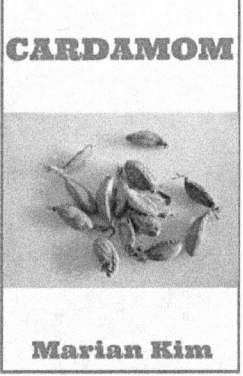

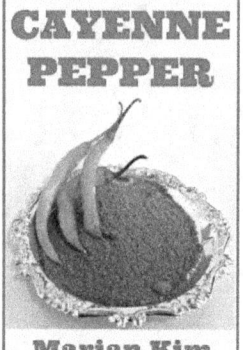

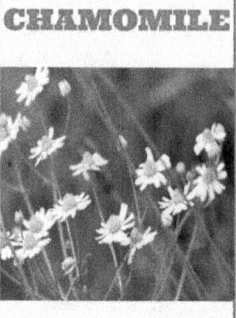

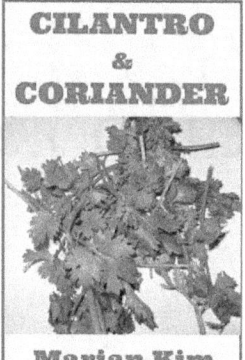

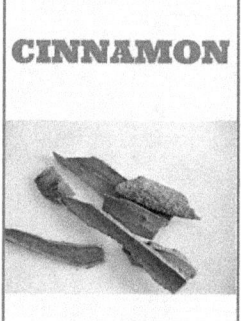

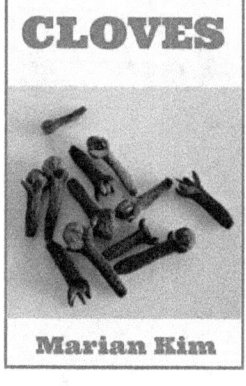

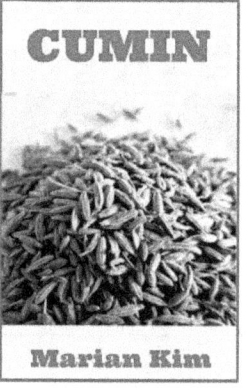

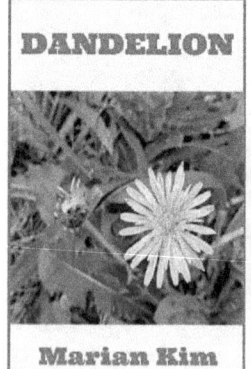

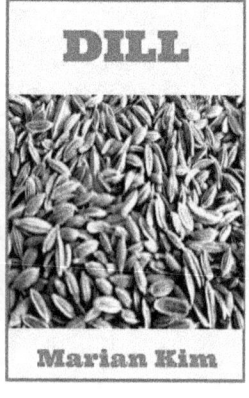

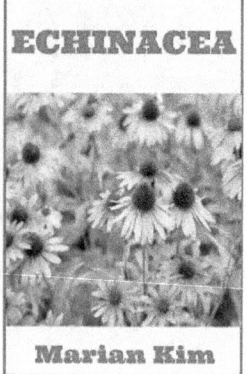

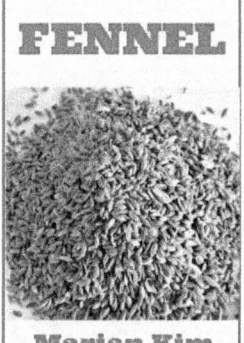

FENNEL

Marian Kim

FENUGREEK

Marian Kim

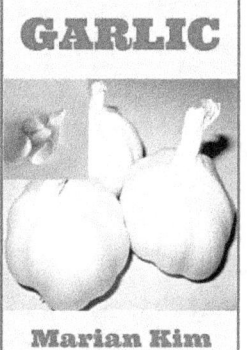

GARLIC

Marian Kim

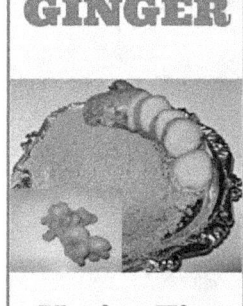

GINGER

Marian Kim

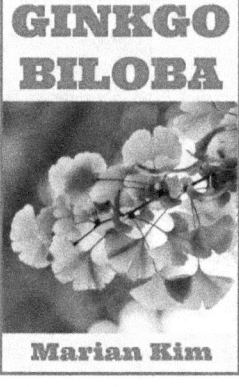

GINKGO BILOBA

Marian Kim

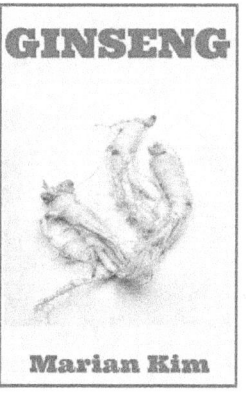

GINSENG

Marian Kim

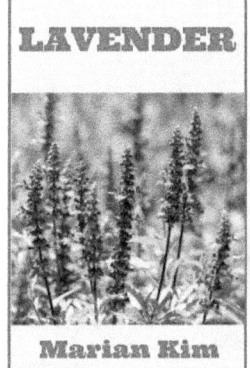

LAVENDER

Marian Kim

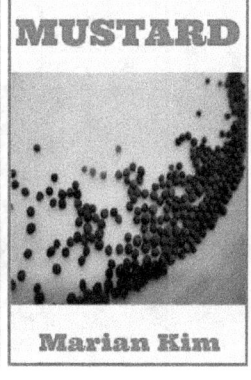

MUSTARD

Marian Kim

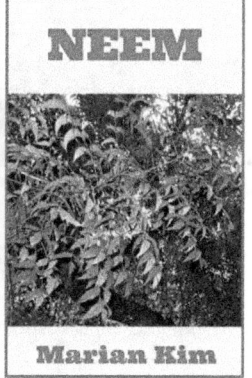

NEEM

Marian Kim

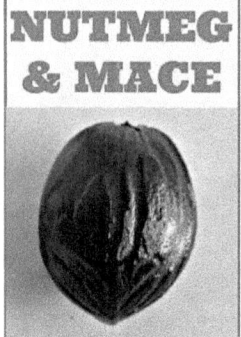

NUTMEG & MACE

Marian Kim

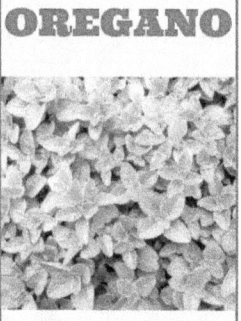

OREGANO

Marian Kim

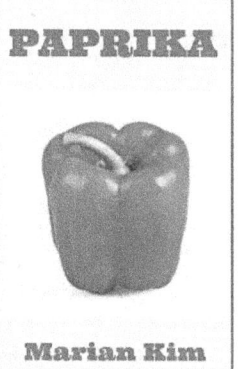

PAPRIKA

Marian Kim

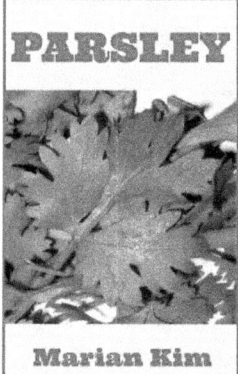

PARSLEY

Marian Kim

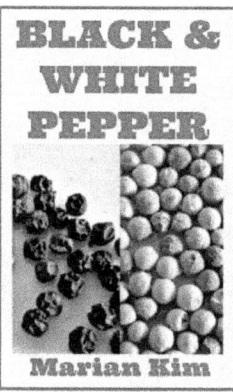

BLACK & WHITE PEPPER

Marian Kim

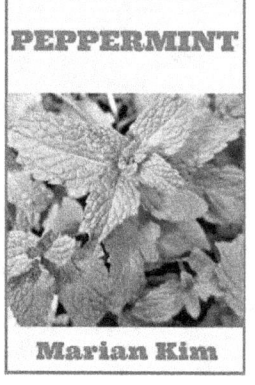

PEPPERMINT

Marian Kim

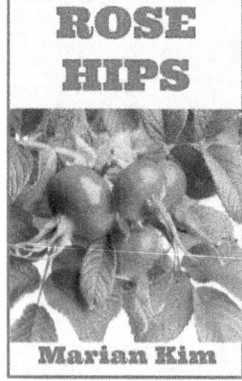

ROSE HIPS

Marian Kim

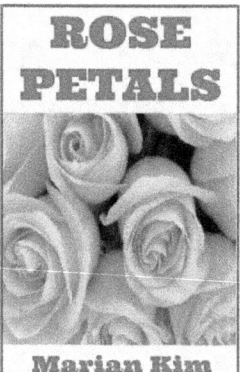

ROSE PETALS

Marian Kim

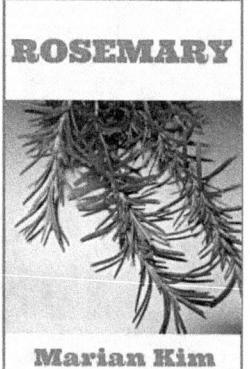

ROSEMARY

Marian Kim

SAGE

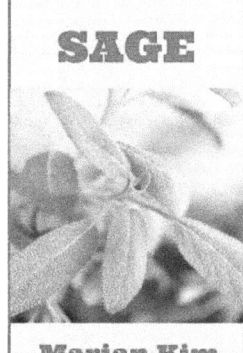

Marian Kim

ST. JOHN'S WORT

Marian Kim

STAR ANISE

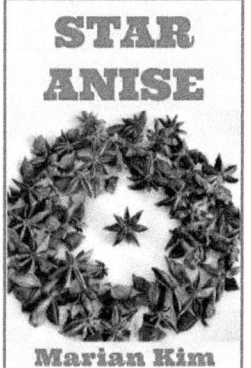

Marian Kim

STINGING NETTLE

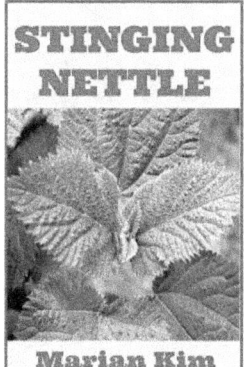

Marian Kim

THYME

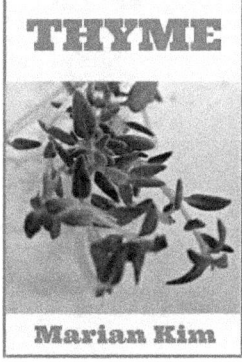

Marian Kim

TURMERIC

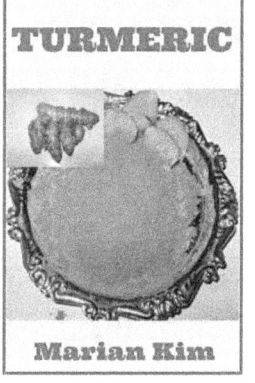

Marian Kim

WITCH HAZEL

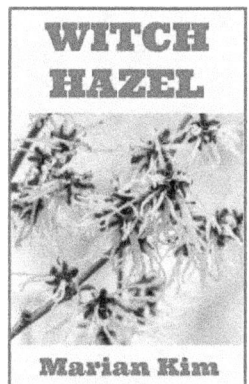

Marian Kim

YARROW

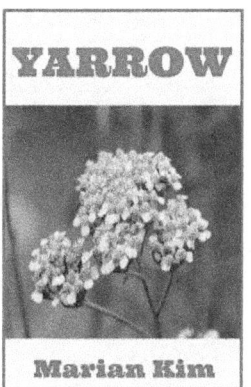

Marian Kim

*****

www.ingramcontent.com/pod-product-compliance
Lightning Source LLC
Chambersburg PA
CBHW070525290526
45790CB00003B/1298